A Journal of One Woman's Spiritual and Wellness Journey Through Covid-19

by

Leslie Romine, R.N., PRS

DORRANCE
PUBLISHING CO
EST. 1920
PITTSBURGH, PENNSYLVANIA 15238

Dorrance Publishing Co
585 Alpha Drive
Pittsburgh, PA 15238
Visit our website at www.dorrancebookstore.com

ISBN: 979-8-88925-123-1
eISBN: 979-8-88925-623-6

This book is dedicated to my mother,
Carmella Ann (COPPOLA) Romine
and my father Lester Marlon Romine.
Thank you for your sacrifice, guidance, wisdom
and unwavering love to me.

February 1st, 2021-

Today. I was inspired to write this journal for all the world. There is no discrimination against race, creed, or socioeconomic statures. Covid hates everyone and wants to take over our bodies, families, friends. All people our lives touch and they touch ours. Whether I die or not, I want this journal to help reach, help, inspire, and heal all affected with this relentless plague and/or have mental health issues they are dealing with.

Since March of last year, all the world started to wake up and see the beginning shock, disbelief, and adaptation of our lives like never before. After 11 months of lockdowns and panic, vaccinations started coming out at a warp speed. Pfizer first, Moderna second, Astra Zeneca, and Johnson and Johnson's last. Unfortunately, J and J's vaccine was only 63% to around 80% effective, while the others were over 90% effective. Both varieties need two shots for ultimate effectiveness. We can still get Covid-19, won't die, but will have mild to moderate illness.

This reflection shows how in our world inequality does not exist with Covid-19, and we should all come together to see this vision. As it is said, God loved his only son, that he gave him to this world to die for our sins.

During Covid-19, in September of 2020, I decided for the first time in my life to seek the advice from a psychiatrist. His name is Dr. Robert E. Ketcham and lives in Virginia. He has been practicing for over 45 years. He is an excellent psychiatrist. He is a great listener and always explains to me what my feelings and actions are displayed in a clear to understand fashion, that sometimes I have trouble discerning. I have consulted with him over the past several years and have grown from all his remarkable advice and education! I highly recommend to anyone who needs great advice and help with anxiety, stress, PTSD, etc. to consult with a psychiatrist and see if they fit into your overall wellness routine as I have.

With Covid-19, there is hope through social distance, masks, and vaccinations. My journal of anxiety and stress as well as working through past PTSD (Post Traumatic Stress) will be uncovered in this book to show resources, living through a pandemic with certain mental health challenges through my daily life, and communication with various organizations for Peer Support and Personal Medicine. LMECC (Laurie Mitchell Empowerment And Career Center) whose website is info@lmec.org, is run by the Inspiring Executive Director Heather Peck. She is a wonderful woman who also is a Certified Peer Support Specialist as well as a Certified Personal Medicine Coach Trainer. She has devoted her life and kindness to helping others through LMECC. They offer Employment Support Services, Peer Support Services, Personal

Medicine Classes, Computer Services, and other resources. Personal Medicine is a class established by the renowned Patricia E. Deegan, Ph.D. She received her PhD in clinical psychology and is the founder of Pat Deegan and Associates (PDA). A great trainer, consultant, and speaker in mental health self-awareness for over 30 years, who I highly respect. A website for her is www.commongroundprogram.com. She is a disability-rights advocate, psychologist, and researcher living in the United States. This wonderful class teaches you to advocate for your own self-care through many teachings' modalities. It is not, as Dr. Pat Deegan says, about "Generic Coping Skills," as it is a way for you to build your own "Powerful Personal Medicine Activities." Per Dr. Pat Deegan, this Personal Medicine class is what we do to get well and stay well. It can be the big things that give our lives meaning and purpose. It can also be the smaller things we do to take care of ourselves. You must take a Certified Personal Medicine Coach training course in order to teach the classes. Work Strategy classes with Marja Lee Freeman, who works with LMECC, is an awesome motivational speaker, employment specialist, and author of the book, "Career Building: How to STAND OUT, Get Ahead and Get Noticed!" Her inquisitive questions make us think about what and why we want a job, and creatively think about interviewing, researching jobs, and how to land a job you really want. Through her psychological questions and employment skills, she helps you feel more confident in finding your new career. Her mission is to empower others to find their destiny. Katey Kerns, Employment Specialist in LMECC's Career Center, worked with me and emailed me several job opportunities. Her main goal is to make sure the jobseeker understands they are not alone, and she is with them during their employment journey and thereafter. Marja Lee Freeman works with us during the second part of a two-hour class with the amazing Sharon Martin who works with DBSA (Depression and Bipolar Support Assistance). She is the Assistant Director and Meetings Coordinator. She is also a Peer Support Specialist. Work website is DBSA of VA.org and personal Gmail is SharonMartinDBSA@yahoo.com. This national organization has been operating for 22 years and is the only one that represents Virginia. It also supports military personnel and government contractors that are deployed overseas. This class gives you so many ways to evaluate your mental health outlook and get to the core of why you think about certain topics; each week she talked about while motivating you during your job search. I found so much happiness, connections, and fulfillment through implementation of all these classes.

These classes I took during the pandemic on Mondays, Tuesdays, and Fridays taught me so many ways of looking at finding a job, remaining resilient, mindful, and extremely hopeful for what the future holds! I implore you to find any class to take and explore the world of Personal Medicine, Peer Support groups, and Work Strategy.

February 1st, 2021—

Today's DBSA/Work Strategy class showed me the utmost value of kindred souls. Zoom, what a funny name for an immensely needed platform to have meetings. All the hosts are amazing and have been serving others throughout their careers. I am so lucky to have met and participated in their class. This ongoing class gave me insights with thinking and working strategies to get ready to find and interview for a job opportunity. Also, DBSA and the Work Strategy class expressed emphatically, never give up! Yesterday and today, we received snow and sleet. I saw pandas playing in the freshly white snow on YouTube at the National Zoo in Washington, D.C. At today's Personal Medicine class, I watched a video that showed a more positive way to make you more mindful and is a gift to inspire the happier moments in our life. We were asked to present a topic to the group on Zoom. I talked about my rendition about a women's view of Covid-19. My thoughts flowed like a waterfall cascading down a beautiful mountain. I sure felt overjoyed being able to connect to other peers and talk about my subject.

Personal Medicine, according to Dr. Pat Deegan, is also a specific activity, not a feeling or state of being. What we do to stay well during life's trials and tribulations. As the wise statement says, "laughter is the best medicine!" Try laughing when things are very stressful and see how you feel. I feel most of the time extremely relieved and my mind refocuses on a happier area. I do this by watching a funny movie, reading funny jokes, or just listening to my friend's jokes.

February 2nd, 2021—

Today, I attended Personal Medicine class about anxiety. I watched the video on Personal Medicine and Physical Health. Personal Medicine is so important now while we all are going through the Covid-19 Pandemic. This video helped me understand how a mental challenge can affect our bodies. I see how important it is to exercise, eat right for our body to function adequately, and not decrease our immune system. Last night, the news reported one case of the Covid-19 variant from South Africa is in Baltimore, Maryland. Luckily, the patient had minor symptoms. When will the worry and anxiety end? My quote today in class was "the man that moves a mountain begins by carrying small stones" by Confucius. How amazingly funny and true is that? It reminds me of the anonymous saying from years ago: "What me Worry?" How simple those days were. We are so lucky to live in the United States and to have modern medicine technology and know this deadly pandemic will not last forever. Laughter is truly a great way to alleviate worry, anxiety, and stress in our lives. When you have lived through PTSD, as I have, any small thing can trigger panic attacks. Praying to God from my bible readings helps to refocus my mind, find peace, and move those little stones to finally overcome that mountain! Today, our weather temperature is 32-33 degrees in Virginia. I am slightly cold but very grateful for the heat in my apartment, clothes on my back, and food in my refrigerator— that's daily gratitude!

I have been taking more online courses and webinars that are helping me educate myself in customer care, mindfulness, finances, and becoming more resilient. All of these are part of my toolbox of Personal Medicine activities. They bring purpose and meaning to me. I have talked to several people from LMECC's Career Center and found educational advice for writing cover letters. I have been utilizing the job search website Indeed to look for various jobs in customer service at a religious organization and healthcare settings. I have been taking computer classes with Amanuel Paulos Ghebremichael, who is LMECC's Educational/Training Program Director and Computer Skills and Digital Literacy Instructor. He is showing me a world into computer skills and digital literacy. I have never ventured into it, and he is a consummate instructor! He instructs not only the workplace productivity tools of Microsoft Office Suites and Google Products but helps you see the concepts related to them. He has an extensive academic background. He is extremely well educated, obtaining a master's degree at George Washington University in Washington, D.C. in International Law.

February 5th, 2021—

Today, I went to a virtual job fair. It was a career fair to listen to employers who do hire people that are older. This was through the wonderful group, SCSEP (The Senior Community Service Employment Program), of which I had been enrolled in as a volunteer, not employee, to gain updated skills: they are affiliated with NCOA (National Council on Aging), instituted through the Federal Government. Also, The Jewish Council on Aging virtual 50 plus virtual job fair I attended today. I have been looking for a remote job, and joining these job fairs shows me what skills are needed to work remotely.

February 9th, 2021—

LMECC Personal Medicine class was about sleep and negative thoughts. Our Personal Medicine Host, Heather Peck, was very helpful, showing us videos and allowing, as she always does give each one of us in the Zoom class time to talk about our Personal Medicine activities we do to stay well and lead a more fulfilling life. The class, as usual, was fun led by her and gave me a lot of wisdom activities from the other participants. The Negative Thoughts video and talks helped uplift my spirits! Covid-19 is still a pandemic, and I am waiting for my age group to get vaccinated.

February 12th, 2021—

The ugly monster comes out—anxiety. I will take small steps to achieve the goal through Personal Medicine. I will work on my specific activities to not be fearful of taking the Covid vaccination. I decided today to utilize two activities: 1. Spell out the pros and cons of the vaccination, and 2. Pray to God for his strength and guidance. In Personal Medicine, these are specific activities that bring a smile to my face and help me feel better about potential reactions to the vaccination because I have had Chronic Idiopathic Urticaria for seven years and might react. Today, in Heather Peck's LMECC's Personal Medicine class, I spoke about this. Because of talking to other peers and feeling so connected, it helped me to continue my journey of this impending topic. Through using these activities daily, it allows me to get well and stay well about my decision to receive the Covid vaccination, take the fear away, and use these small steps to clear my mind of self-doubt. I felt so much better after practicing these wellness activities for several days! I analyzed what is the worst-case scenario, the best-case scenario, and what will likely happen. And with the grace of God in my life, I prepared ahead to structure this situation into a positive outcome! It is 4:23 p.m. and I feel more relaxed, less anxious, and happy about my situation after I took a walk around my neighborhood.

February 16th, 2021—

There is a virtual job fair for people over 50 years old that I will be attending. I am excited about this. Yesterday, which was a Monday, I was bored except for my friend's company and support. I am still waiting to get a vaccination. The two most contagious strains now are in Virginia now: 1. UK variant, and 2. African variant. The CDC recommends we double up our masks. The job fair lasted from ten to two p.m. I am glad I participated via Zoom even though I did not get the response I would have liked from certain employers. Not a lot of employers are hiring remotely. Tonight at six p.m., I have a webinar on Extreme Customer Service Skills, and tomorrow at noon, I have a webinar on Upskilling for Talented Workers. These webinars are free and great to attend. Anyone can find an email for your city or county that offers all kinds of different webinars. If you participate in the SCSEP program, you will receive listings as well as other info pertinent to share.

February 22, 2021—

I am feeling very joyful and grateful for my life, and my loved ones in my life. Life is so amazing. Every day is a NEW BEGINNING! I pray in the morning and thank God for what he has given me and for protection during the day. I have been dealing with a strained muscle in my left lower back since Feb. 14th. This has increased my anxiety and I asked myself: "How did this happen? Did I lift too many heavy waters or was it exercising?" When it started it was very painful and hard to get up from my couch or chairs. I can't take much Motrin because of my Urticaria. I made an appointment to see my internal medicine doctor on the 17th and he diagnosed me with a muscle spasm and prescribed a muscle relaxer as well as for me to continue with using my heating pad. Within two days, I started to feel so much better, less pain, and my mobility was coming back. Thank God for modern medicine, great medicines, and great doctors.

Today, Covid-19 update: the UK variant is in of our 50 states. Last week, a 65-year-old man in Maryland died from the African variant. I will get my vaccination to protect me as well as others form this horrible virus! I mentally thought about my wellness activity today. I decided today to weigh the pros—build up my antibodies so

I have less chance of dying from Covid-19 and cons—I may react se-verely with my Chronic Urticaria or mildly, a couple of days of mild to moderate itching and non-invasive mild hives. My allergist/im-munologist doctor believes I won't react badly. I prayed to God and left this mountain of unknowns to him: another Personal Medicine tool, and immediately, I felt a sense of overall peace and happiness!

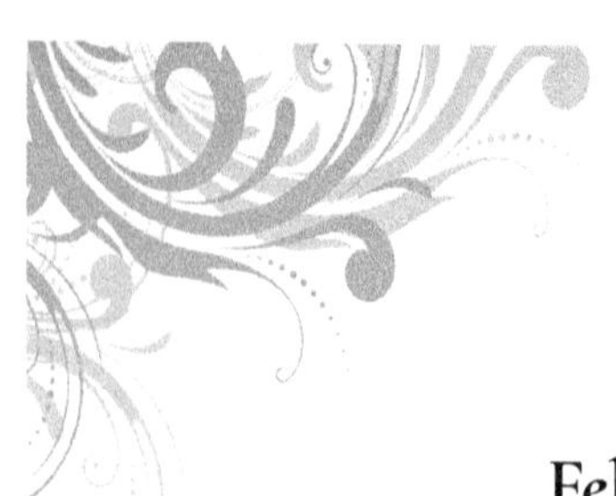

February 26th, 2021—

Today, I feel sad because my Chronic Urticaria is very bad. I am itching all over my body. I pray every morning and ask God for his help to get me through the day. I thank him for my blessings and that I will be a positive influence in someone's life today.

My best friend is getting his vaccination today—hurray! I prayed for him to be alright. He said the second one sometimes is worse than the first, but it is different how everyone reacts. While I waited to hear how it went, I wrote in my journal. This activity helps me redirect my mind and is one way I keep busy. It is an activity in my Personal Medicine that helps me keep busy and relieve my mind's thoughts.

I pray for all the abused, mentally challenged, homeless, hungry women, men, and animals to be made happy and healthy. For all the people over the world who have died or are very sick from Covid-19, I pray for your souls and suffering you have endured.

March 9th, 2021—

Today, my LMECC Personal Medicine class focused on Negative Thinking. This session really helped me with my negative thoughts. I will call on my higher power and replace negative thoughts with gratitude for the good things in my life. This changes and redirects my mind to a positive outlook. These activities sustain my outlook on my daily life, uplift me to a positive mindset and lessen my anxiety. I am finally registered for my Covid-19 vaccination. I can't wait to receive this shot and get my body to produce antibodies against this heinous virus. I am looking forward to receiving from the Johnson and Johnson vaccine 65-73% immunity. My anxieties and PTSD through this pandemic and other life issues have been diminishing through the help of DBSA/Work Strategy Group and Personal Medicine classes with LMECC! I have found there is nothing better than human interaction, even if it is in a Zoom class. I have strengthened my relationship with Jesus Christ and feel so much stronger. I pray daily for his love, forgiveness, and protection.

March 15, 2021—

Today, I feel alone. I had conversations with a peer group last Friday and shared my insights. Why is it so hard to find a part-time job? I believe through careful education it is ageism. How horrible that topic is because I have so much more wisdom, responsibility, and discipline. My best friends will be contacted, and I will share my thoughts. I enjoy talking with Josh about this and he will be with me in the evening after I receive my vaccination. My other best friend, Andy, will be with me during the vaccination. We often play checkers. After studying his tactics, I am becoming quite good at this game. Like life, the game changes every time we play, and it forces me to strategize while playing to win. On Sunday, I received a text from my doctor's office that I am still on a waiting list to receive the shot.

Daily, I struggle with living alone and if I structure my day and keep busy, I feel a sense of great meaning and structure in my life. At night it gets hard sometimes being alone. I am learning to also have a routine to combat that. This was not an issue until the pandemic struck us all. My anxiety and stress levels have been minimal at this time.

Last Sunday, I went to church with a mask on and had a joyous time. When I received the Eucharist, it tasted so good—like honey!

What a great Personal Medicine for me. Usually, I always watch my Catholic Mass and other religious shows on the television. This mass resounded with me spot on and I love being a Christian.

March 21st, 2021—

I am still waiting to get my vaccination. My thoughts are positive, and ready to get this shot. I now see the positive and have addressed the problem-solving worries of this. God is with me and in control. It is a relief psychologically to realize there are many things I can't control. As T.D. Jakes wrote, "Don't allow your past or present condition to control you. It is just a process you are going through to get to the next level." I focus on God and inspirational quotes to reaffirm my wisdom and resiliency and take my life one day at a time. I have seen throughout this pandemic when one door closes, another door opens. That excites me to remain always curious about what will happen next.

March 28th, 2021—

I am getting my J and J shot on March 30th. I am excited and anxious at the same time. I catch myself acting in a giddy manner. Praying to God is so helpful now. I will be so elated to get this finally done. I read that J and J is coming out with a booster shot. I am so happy about this. I chose to go with this shot first to see how my body responds, then take Moderna's vaccination down the road. My best friend, Andy, is going with me to the doctor's office and will stay with me for several hours to watch for any anaphylactic reaction. My other best friend, Josh, will stay the night with me. We have our game plan, and I will enjoy both of their company. Andy and Josh are both very good people that I have known for about twenty years. They are wonderful to talk with and watch over me. I am very blessed; I have a great support system. I have also spoken to my brother as well.

March 30th, 2021—

It is 8:28 a.m.; today is the day to get my shot. I am so happy to give back something else to protect society against Covid-19. I am excited to get this over with, and can't wait to get the next booster shot that will increase my antibody's level even higher to help keep me out of a hospital or even die if I caught Covid-19. I have prayed that everyone all over the world who will get this vaccination has the adequate supplies of shots to do so.

I received my shot at 1:30 p.m. from a Physician's Assistant (PA), I have some redness (pruritis), but no severe reaction and it is nine p.m.! Thank you, God, for your positive blessing of your protection. I am so happy! My stress and anxiety level have decreased by 50%. Sometimes, a delayed reaction can occur, so I will see what tomorrow brings.

March 31st, 2021—

Twenty-four hours later, postshot. I have a slightly sore arm and mild to moderate itching. I do feel dehydrated, so I am drinking more water. I am not fatigued, feeling ill or depressed! Good Friday is this coming Friday April 2nd. I am praying about Jesus Christ, his passion and fate for all of us. Through my thoughts about my Personal Medicine classes on Zoom I have taken, I feel stronger and happier than ever. My anxiety and PTSD are moderate to minimal, depending on the day.

April 1st, 2021—

After forty-eight hours later, post-shot, my mind feels giddy. How funny that is. Is it because I faced a hurdle and achieved the goal, or is it something else? It is amazing how this vaccine biologically and mentally affects your body. By April 28th, I will have full antibody production at 86% effective against a severe or fatal outcome. I will have 77% antibody effectiveness against a mild to moderate case of Covid.

April 2nd, 2021—

It is truly great to be vaccinated. I am so glad I rushed to get it. I still and will for several years wear an N-95 mask while shopping or in closed environments, even after all the vaccines are given to me. I believe, this virus, since it is replicating, is not going away anytime soon.

April 2nd, 2021—

Seventy-two hours post vaccination and no bad reactions. Thank you, God! Today is Good Friday and I am very solemn. Sunday is Easter or as I say, Resurrection Day! Thank you, God, for sending your son to take away our sins and lead us into eternity with you. It does bother me how they brutalized Jesus. What was he feeling before Judas betrayed him and he was arrested? He already knew what would happen. He must have been so anxious and stressed, knowing his crucifixion was imminent. He did this for us all. This was his path on our Earth to live out, and he went through it with such dignity!

April 6th, 2021—

It is so great to be vaccinated. I am glad I got it quickly. I ponder on how I have felt the last two days. I have felt anxiety and dread, but I don't know why. Maybe it is because the last two days I have had bad dreams. Last night, I dreamt I married an ex-boyfriend, but his friends would not accept my religion. Both of us admitted we could not take the constant negative remarks, so he made the weak decision to separate. The night before that, I dreamt of large white snakes all around me; it was strange and dangerous. I am not sure why these dreams happen; I have read it is our subconscious or possibly something we watched on television the night before that triggered this. I looked up the symbolism and it was a positive/negative connotation. It means purity, energy, and new beginnings. Also, it means something in my life is out of control: hidden threats and/or betrayal. Biblically, it means disappointment and taste of bitterness or betrayal. I decided to remain strong and practice my Personal Medicine activities that make me feel positive and strong. I visualize my heart being pure because good and pure hearts will achieve victory over evil hearts! I also practiced compassion and empathy in my life by listening to my loved ones and helping them through a bad situation they are going through.

April 12th, 2021—

Today, I feel very happy to God for getting me through last night. I watched mass on the television and took the Eucharist during the Catholic Mass I watched. Jesus, I trust in you! I have been praying more and realize during this pandemic and being alone during this unprecedented time, that life is what you make of it. You have good days, and you have bad days. If we can accept this, not fight it, and be compassionate with ourselves, we are progressing forward. To move those little stones, it takes time. Little by little, the stones are removed, and our life seems to flow more easily. Life is a learning experience that is very wonderous and eye opening. What I have realized is that life is a journey where you never stop learning something new, so enjoy the process! That is what my life's ongoing wellness journey is all about.

Through living alone, I have had a lot of time to get to know Jesus better. I believe we are all here to help one another through motivation and compassion. During the good times, we are here to be part of another's special moment, to be happy for them and celebrate their achievement. My Zoom sessions have greatly helped me lessen my anxiety. I feel much more resilient, mindful, and strong after one year of this Covid-19 Pandemic. My Peer Support sessions that involve Personal Medicine have helped me see life in a more positive way. I would recommend anyone who has anxiety or mental challenges in their life to join one.

Today, I am looking forward to my other class I take—DBSA/ Work Strategy. This class keeps me engaged in thinking about how I feel about the topics brought up and work through it. I still have not found a job yet. It is stated that for every one applicant, there are 250-300 applicants! That is mind-blowing. Gone are the good old days of finding a job where there is less competition.

April 14th, 2021—

The FDA is halting the Johnson and Johnson vaccination for now. Six people developed a rare blood clotting disorder. This is six people out of one million vaccinated. To err on caution, the FDA decided to stop and investigate why this has occurred. There has been the same situation with Astra Zeneca. The recipient's presented with this disorder within eight to thirteen days. Today is my fifteenth day after my shot and I have not had any occurrence of clots.

April 17th, 2021—

I feel very strong and resilient today. Through Jesus's grace, I have endured this pandemic. I look forward to seeing what is going to happen next in my life. Some areas in Virginia and Maryland are experiencing shortages of the vaccines. I empathize with the people waiting to receive the shot. I have been reading my journal today, and I have experienced all the anger, fear, shock and worry in my daily life. I feel now from reading my journal to publish it so I can reach others who have lived through this time and have had mental health challenges and feelings like me. If I can help anyone and show just one person how to master common mental challenges and lead a stronger, more eye-opening, and fulfilled life, that is my ultimate happiness goal!

April 22nd, 2021—

My Personal Medicine activity today is my mantra that I will repeat many times today: I am a visionary, creative, resilient, and very empathetic, strong woman! This made me feel joyful and content. I found out today that Johnson and Johnson vaccine will be cleared this Friday, April 24th, by the CDC. I am not concerned about the side-effects of the blood clotting disorder. They found women from the age of 18-48 years old is the target area of concern. They found so far that they had low platelet counts and some had prior use of Heparin, which is an anti-coagulant medicine. I have seen in the news that there are so many people in the United States, who are not willing to get the vaccination.

I feel so much growth in myself since February 1st, 2021, when I started my journal. Journaling helps your mind to focus on something that is important to you. It is one of my Personal Medicine activities that puts a smile on my face. It lets me let go of any stressful thoughts I am experiencing. Expressing my mind on paper is very liberating for me because it also allows me to feel a purpose and meaning in my life. My life has a stronger and quicker way to bounce back from a negative situation. How liberating! It makes me zone out to the state of mindfulness; this is the art of living in the moment and all outside occurrences take a second seat. Mindfulness comes in many forms I have utilized: taking walks and just looking at the trees, hearing the birds chirping, or seeing the houses around me, listening to soft music, watching a funny movie, or praying. This is another way I get through the pandemic, or any strife in life that may happen daily. I hope you try this and see for yourself how it can alleviate stress, anxiety, and depression.

May 6th, 2021—

I have begun to feel that my life's purpose has diminished. In the past three mornings, it has been hard for me to wake up and feel excited about my purpose for the day. The news last night said there are less jobs than before the pandemic. After several days, I decided to focus on the positive sides of my life. I am journaling and it has filled a void, I have wonderful, loved ones that are always there for me, and I know God will take care of the rest. I remember the Serenity Prayer and I will stay a resilient and creative thinker! I continue to access LinkedIn's job alerts and other job search vehicles.

May 24th, 2021—

Covid cases are dropping! Vaccinations are working to slow this insidious virus. I am feeling so elated at this news. Restrictions are being lifted. Slowly, life in the United States is returning to a "New Normal." I am still investigating job listings to find a comparable fit to my circumstances. I look forward to a new opportunity that I can use my wisdom and life work skills.

June 16th, 2021—

I was scammed on a social networking site for a job. I told the person who I connected with to cease all communication with me. I did not give out any personal or financial information, nor would I, because that is always a red flag. I was told a long time ago about the potential for scammers and fraudulent people. On any website, you connect to you must always be very vigilant.

People are still getting sick from the Covid-19 virus, and it makes me feel sadness and great compassion for them. A lot of people refuse to get vaccinated. There have been so many deaths from this horrible virus. India is still ranking high number of cases. They have not received enough vaccinations for the enormous population there. Why does this have to be? What is wrong with our humanity?

June 18th, 2021—

This day is starting out rough for me. I feel anxious. I dwell on the fact that I cannot eat the type of foods I ate eight years ago because of reactions with my Chronic Urticaria. I will review one of my Personal Medicine cards to help me work through this problem. While working on my solution, it dawned on me how many good things I have in my life. I feel very blessed by God because I have had many magical moments. I will practice gratitude for what I have in my life now and compassion for others with this illness or who just should have compassion given to them. Also, I will pray for God's healing power. These reflections help me to divert my mindset from a gloomy to positive mood.

Unfortunately, another dilemma with my right posterior tendon, of which I have a permanent partial tear has flared up and I have been icing it for the past two days. It is about 90% better. Staying off it always helps it to get better as well.

July 5th, 2021—

I feel happy and peaceful. The sun is out, my body feels strong, God is with me and all my friends, family, and loved ones are healthy. Throughout this Covid-19 period, I keep seeing the strength of resilience, gratitude, and compassion that has lifted my spirit, increased my mature growth, and opened a new world to me. This new world emphasizes how much better I feel when I can assist and help others that are suffering or want advice during a crisis or just everyday stresses in life.

There is a Delta variant of Covid-19 in the fifty states of the United States. It started in India, because sadly, they have not received enough vaccinations fast enough, so Covid will keep replicating these new variants for a long while. I always wear a mask and do not want to be in large groups yet. Even if you are vaccinated, there is the potential you can still catch it, and no one knows the very long consequences to our bodies.

July 23rd, 2021—

The Delta variant is roaring through the United States at an alarming pace. The unvaccinated and even vaccinated people are catching it. Many vaccinated or unvaccinated people don't wear their masks. The United Kingdom and other parts of Europe are infected with the new variant.

Break through cases are increasing, and Pfizer and Johnson and Johnson are working on a booster shot. I will get the Johnson and Johnson booster shot when it is available. There is no definite data percentage on the Johnson and Johnson vaccine, but their officials say it is 60% effective against the Delta variant, and Pfizer is 66-74% effective.

California increase in Covid-19 infections has increased so much that the mayor has instituted all vaccinated and non-vaccinated people to wear a mask indoors in any retail or restaurant business. They were a couple of weeks ago where Virginia is now.

I think we should mandate mask wearing as well. There have been 383 new cases of the Delta variant since yesterday, and hospitals have admitted mostly unvaccinated patients as well as some vaccinated by 66% as of yesterday.

I am not eating inside restaurants, unless it is sparsely filled with one or two couples, or I will pick up my food to go, because a lot of waiter and waitresses do not wear masks.

This new variant originally spread from India, who still does not have ample amounts of the vaccination to help those who want to be vaccinated.

Unfortunately, another variant, Lambda is around the corner. I am praying for all those dying and those becoming sick from this virus all round this Earth. It is hard to watch the news of the people in hospitals who are very sick and will potentially die from this Covid-19 and its variants or read about it. It is also hard for me to know people who are not getting vaccinated and not wearing a mask. This Covid-19 replicates and mutates like no other virus I have seen in the past. Anyone can get it and pass it to another who could have life-threatening circumstances.

July 27th, 2021—

Many states and counties in the United States are mandating workers in various fields to get vaccinated or have weekly tests for the virus. In Los Angeles, California, they have mandated mask wearing in stores and other businesses. Virginia is asking people to get vaccinated because of the contagious Delta variant. I pray that people will hear this message and get vaccinated. The long-term aftereffects of Covid-19 are not very well known. Some people so far that caught the virus have had long-term brain fog, fatigue, and loss of smell and taste.

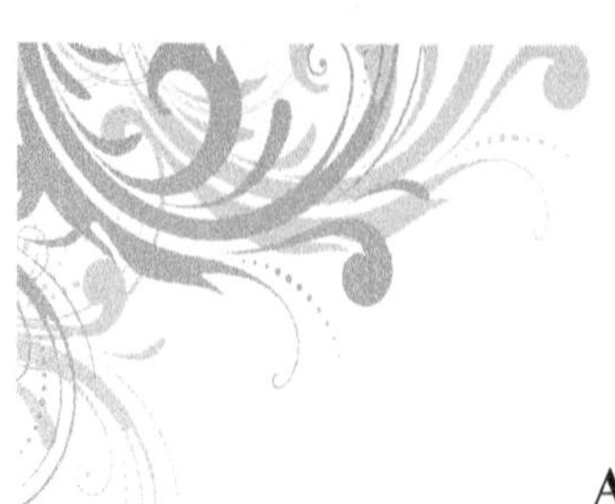

August 2nd, 2021—

It baffles me that many people are not wearing a mask. It saddens me that people are tired of this pandemic and do not want to keep changing their life and be vigilant about precautions. I saw a show on the television about nurses who did not want to get the vaccination. I know that we all have the right to not get vaccinated, but why take the chance? They did not ask any of the nurses if they cared for any Covid patients.

I feel humbled to feel God's presence in my life. It keeps me resilient and strong to pray and be grateful none of my loved ones have become sick; this is a very powerful Personal Medicine to me. I feel so lucky to be born in the United States of America. Colonists fought to establish and build our United States. They suffered, died, fought, and endured many hardships to lay the foundation of this great nation. So, I wonder, if we think about that, why can't we live in a new normal, mask up, keep our guard up, practice safe habits, and learn to give up a couple of years to get through the worst of this virus?

August 2nd, 2021—

What I have learned about myself from August 2020 to August 2021: all people deserve compassion, and all nations should band together to eradicate this virus and its non-ending variants. I will stay connected through Personal Medicine classes. Take courses that are free and teach me new skills, especially coaches who help teach me how to develop and work through my mental health challenges. Further practice being in a state of mindfulness. Continue learning how to be better at remaining flexible to another's thoughts, communicating effectively, and practicing patience. Pick your friends wisely. I believe good friends are those who you give 100% to, and they counter you with a 100% positive friendship. I don't watch news that is constantly negative and can trigger negative thoughts within me. Keep your goals in mind for reviewing where you are at in three, six, and nine months. If I feel isolated in between various activities during my day, or stalled in my life, I will remember to take it one day at a time and see what each week renders to me. Lastly, plan your day; write down what you want to accomplish daily and weekly. This always helps me to structure my day and have a purpose driven outcome. At nighttime, I will feel grateful and name what I am grateful for, and I will try to help give sound advice to my friends who desire it.

Since April 2nd, 2021, more Delta variants have been reported in the United States. The Federal Government has mandated as before, masks to be worn in several buildings, schools, etc. I am thankful for all the sound health advice, friends, family, peer groups, Personal Medicine, and prayer to get me through this trying time. Prayer has helped me strengthen my resiliency, connection to God, and lead a more healthy and mindful life.

December 2021—

A new variant has emerged from South Africa. It is called Omicron. The CDC is asking all Americans to make sure we are vaccinated, wear masks, social distance, and use much care in social gatherings.

January 25th, 2022—

The Omicron variant now comprises 98% of cases in the United States. There are very high cases of this variant in the United Kingdom, Europe, and the rest of this world. The good news is the variant is less severe and there are less deaths or severe cases among the vaccinated.

On November 3rd, 2021, I received my second dose of the Johnson and Johnson vaccination. I had three days of itching and pruritis. My allergist/immunologist doctor stated that is a good sign to show that it is working. My doctor ordered an antigen blood test in December, to see what my level was for fighting Covid-19 and other variants. It was 190, which is high and great for my body to fight any breakthough infection of the Covid-19 or other variants, because antibodies are growing from the vaccinations.

The news has stated that the cases are getting better, and the WHO (World Health Organization), believes the number of cases will calm down soon. This seems to be correlated from the amount of people all over our world being vaccinated. I feel empowered by God, our medicine knowledge and my family, friends, and loved ones who have not caught this original or new variants of the original virus.

April 11, 2022—

Today, I have been thinking about finishing my journal which I always wanted to turn into a book to help inspire others. I realize and accept this is the new normal I must get used to and thrive. Each day I have seen information about the Covid-19 variants, trends of death cases, self-survival tactics, and being aware of how we protect ourselves each day in our lives.

This Friday is the day when Jesus Christ was crucified. And I am reminded of his life preceding his death and then his resurrection. How he dealt with his impending death and how he still brought compassion and strength to others. I realize that the challenges I have faced in the past have made me learn more about myself. It has shown me that I have grown. It took a lot of strength for me to look within myself, face the challenges I have been grappling with, and then discern how to handle, educate, connect more, and live with it in my daily life. I am very happy with my results so far. I realize that my life is a journey of learning, connecting, and practicing certain Personal Medicine activities that are powerful for me. As a Catholic, I see how this parallels Jesus Christ's life. This is a reminder for all of us who have experienced great stress, anxiety, PTSD, or depression.

Praying is powerful for me. It contents me, relieves my burdens, and helps me achieve a closer bond to God.

August 1st, 2022—

A new variant of concern is BA.2 and BA.5 after the Omicron variant. I have been vaccinated twice with Johnson and Johnson shots and, the Moderna booster vaccination as well. Moderna has another booster vaccination coming out in the fall to add these new variants. This booster will be called the bivalent booster. I am eagerly anticipating it. On Monday only, I was placed in a volunteer training site through The Skill Source, which is affiliated with SCSEP/NCOA, for only four hours. I am always wearing a mask.

So, this is the new normal. Masks, washing hands, new vaccinations, being careful in restaurants and in social gatherings. Being ready for any newer variants that keep emerging.

Conclusion—

I hope my journal of my spiritual and wellness journey through this dreadful pandemic with Covid-19 will help you. Writing this journal and looking back through my entries sparked me to publish it to show how any person with daily mental health challenges can grow and change you to live a happier and more fulfilling life. Anyone with any issue can benefit by connecting to a Peer Recovery Group, Personal Medicine Group, taking classes to put your mind in a peaceful state or connecting with a psychologist, psychiatrist, therapist, coach, or mentor. I mentioned earlier that there are career development and personal development resources you can reach out to as well. You can always call a hot line if you are experiencing a crisis and you can consult a doctor to see if you need medications to get you through your medical diagnosis.

Whether you struggle with stress, anxiety, PTSD, depression, other mental health challenges or just need a boost in your life, these resources I listed are wonderful ways to connect, share with others who are going through the same thing. Connection is so important to the healing and growth process in our lives. These helped me to become more mindful, resilient, and have more compassion for myself and to feel always hopeful for the future. Give yourself a big pat on your back, you made it through another pandemic day! These resources are a fabulous way to help you with your strife's in your life's journey! I wish all my readers all the Best of Good Mental Health and Joy in your lives!

In conclusion, I have four questions to ask you:
1. What feelings did you experience when Covid-19 began?
2. What did you do mentally, physically, emotionally, and spiritually to help you get through your day with these feelings?
3. What have you learned about yourself during the pandemic?
4. Do you feel stronger, more resilient, and compassionate toward yourself and others?

www.ingramcontent.com/pod-product-compliance
Lightning Source LLC
Chambersburg PA
CBHW061642130726
47996CB00003B/1417